The 25,000 Mark:
It's Not Just a Concussion

The 25,000 Mark:
It's Not Just A Concussion

Kelli A. Uitenham CScD, SLP-CCC, CBIS

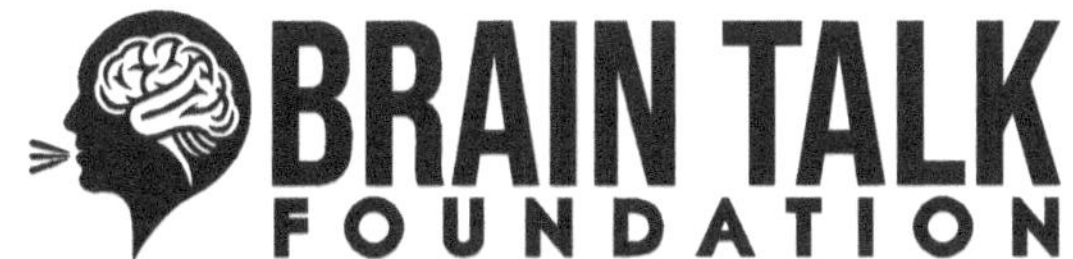

Copyright © 2026 by Brain Talk Foundation

All rights reserved.

No part of this book may be reproduced, distributed, or transmitted in any form or by any means, including photocopying, recording, or other electronic or mechanical methods, without the prior written permission of Brain Talk Foundation, except in the case of brief quotations used in reviews or scholarly works.

Written by Dr. Kelli Uitenham, CCC-SLP, CBIS

Published by Blue Topaz Publishing

Interior design by S.E. Barnabus + Co

Author Photos by DwaShawn The Photographer

Brain Talk Foundation retains all rights to this work.

Print ISBN: 978-1-7325476-7-4

eBook ISBN: 978-1-7325476-6-7

For more information, visit: braintalkfoundation.org
Contact: info@braintalkfoundation.org

Disclaimer: This book is for informational purposes only and is not intended as medical or professional advice. Readers are encouraged to seek appropriate professional support for their individual needs.

Dedication

This book is dedicated to the athletes still taking hits toward the 25,000 mark, those who have already reached it, and those we have lost too soon to CTE. Each of your stories matters.

To the coaches, who choose safety over silence, and to the parents who advocate, protect, and stand in the gap for their children when it matters most.

To the families, who have lost their athletes to CTE, I honor your strength, your courage, and your willingness to share your truth so that others may be protected.

To every reader, what you are about to learn cannot be unlearned. Once you know, you carry a responsibility. Raise awareness by taking this knowledge into your conversations, your communities, and your decisions. Change happens one conversation at a time.

Once you know, what you do next is up to you.
Do with this information what you will.

~ Dr. Kelli ~

Table of Contents

In one of the earliest widely cited studies from Boston University's CTE Center, 110 of 111 former NFL players examined showed evidence of chronic traumatic encephalopathy (CTE).

While this group was not representative of all athletes, the findings sparked a shift in how we understand the long-term effects of repetitive brain injury.

Author's Note:
Why 25,000?

The title *The 25,000 Mark* is inspired by a haunting metaphor used by Dr. Bennet Omalu, the forensic pathologist who first discovered Chronic Traumatic Encephalopathy (CTE) in the brain of NFL Hall of Famer Mike Webster. Webster, a legendary center for the Pittsburgh Steelers, suffered from severe cognitive decline, depression, and dementia after his football career ended. In 2002, when Dr. Omalu examined Webster's brain, he described its condition as being equivalent to someone who had survived 25,000 car crashes.

That number is symbolic. No one knows the precise number of hits it takes for an individual to develop CTE. The risk depends on age, genetics, the force and frequency of impacts, and whether the brain is given time to heal. But the metaphor matters, because it points to the unseen cost of repeated head trauma. Especially in youth athletes, those hits can accumulate silently, long before anyone sees the damage.

In this story, the 25,000 mark represents a threshold, as well as a warning, a wake-up call, and a challenge. It is not a diagnosis. It's a question: how many hits is too many? And what choices will we make before someone reaches that point?

Brett Taylor's journey explores that threshold. The story you're about to read is fictional, but the stakes are very real.

Prologue

The first hit doesn't feel like anything. Just a bump. A jolt. A quick buzz behind the eyes that fades before the next play is even called. No one notices. Not the player. Not the coach. Not the crowd.

Then comes another. And another. And another. Helmet to helmet. Ground to skull. Whiplash. Rattle. Reset. Over time, the body learns to absorb it. The brain just tries to keep up.

Sometimes there's a headache. Sometimes there's a mood. Sometimes there's a forgotten assignment or a short fuse or a night that ends in tears for no clear reason. But there's always a reason. It just takes too long to find it. And by then, the damage has already started.

And no one's keeping score. Not of the hits that don't knock you out. Not of the ones you "shake off." Not of the quiet changes happening inside your mind.

This story is about those hits. The ones that don't make the highlight reel. The ones that build up, bit by bit, until something shifts.

It's about a young man who loved football and who built his

world around it. And what happened when he found himself at a crossroads: to stay silent and stay the course, or to speak up, choose himself, and risk disappointing everyone who believed toughness meant pushing through. His coach. His teammates. His father.

This is the story of what it means to make the hardest call of all. The call to protect your future.

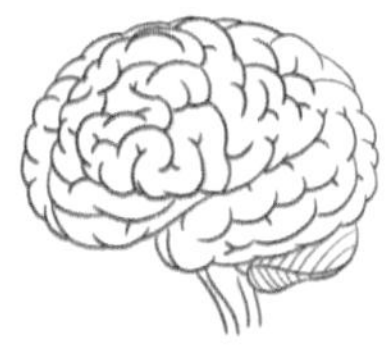

Chapter 1
Friday Night Lights

Brett

Brett jogged onto the field, turf springy beneath his cleats, the stadium lights flaring to life like a second sunrise. The crowd roared, parents, classmates, scouts, all blurring together in a sea of noise. He bounced on the balls of his feet, tugging at his chinstrap like it might keep his heart from punching through his chest.

His first varsity start. Finally. He'd spent three years waiting for this, watching from the sidelines, dreaming in slow motion. Tonight, he had to show them, show himself, that he belonged out here.

"Trips right, 36 power on one! Ready—break!"

The quarterback's voice cut through the static in his head. Brett crouched low, breath tight in his ribs.

Crack.

The collision rang through his helmet like a bell struck too hard. The sky lurched. For a second, the field blurred sideways.

He blinked hard.

Don't say anything. Don't look hurt.

If Coach thought he was out of it, he'd bench him.
If Mom saw, she'd panic. If anyone saw...

This could be my only shot.

His legs moved like they belonged to someone else as he jogged back to the huddle, everything about him pretending to be fine.

The next play snapped before his breath caught up. He lowered his shoulder…another hit, but this one was deeper, like it reached through skin into bone. A wall of muscle folded around him. The sound inside his helmet was all ringing.

The sky was still sideways.

Still, he ran. Sort of.

Shake it off. Don't let them see. Don't give them a reason to pull you.

But something was wrong.

He couldn't feel the play anymore. Just the noise. The tilt. His own body was moving half a second behind his mind.

The Parentals

Angela leaned forward with her hands pressed flat against her thighs. She cheered when the crowd did, but her eyes were locked on her son.

She'd watched enough games to know the rhythm. Angela knew when it flowed clean and when something cracked underneath.

She saw Brett stumble. Just for a moment.

Her hand flew to her mouth.

"Did you see that?" she whispered, grabbing her husband Marcus' arm.

Marcus didn't flinch. The ex-linebacker and college legend. He watched the same play through a different lens.

"It's football babe," he said. "He's fine."

Angela wanted to believe him. She wanted his calm to seep into the places she couldn't steady herself. But something in Brett's body looked…off. She'd know that look anywhere.

"I know my kid," she said under her breath. "Something's not right."

Marcus kept his eyes on the field.

Back in his day, you didn't come out unless you couldn't stand.

Coach Daniels

Coach Daniels slapped Brett's shoulder pads as he jogged to the sideline.

"That's what I'm talkin' about, Taylor! You keep hittin' like that and they'll remember your name."

But even as the words left his mouth, his eyes narrowed.

Brett's focus was off. There was a beat, just a beat, before he responded. A flicker of disconnection.

Daniels had seen it before. He'd pulled kids before. He'd also had angry parents in his office, booster calls lighting up his phone, and the athletic director reminding him what a losing record did to funding.

He glanced toward the stands.

Marcus was watching. Tough-as-nails Marcus. If Daniels pulled his son now…

His hand twitched toward Brett. Then dropped.

"He's fine," he muttered to himself.

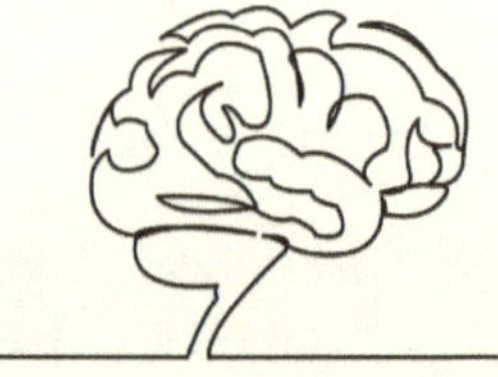

Invisible Symptoms (Unspoken)

Brett's legs wobbled as he took his place on the line again.

Headache.
Like his skull had shrunk two sizes too small.

Confusion.
The play call was a whisper he couldn't quite catch.

Clumsiness.
His left foot caught the turf like it didn't remember how to run.

Sensitivity.
Everything felt too loud, too fast, too bright.

Just keep going. Don't let them see.

Timeout: Reflection

Three people watched the same play unfold.

> **Brett:** Riding the edge of consciousness but refusing to let go.
>
> **Angela:** Heart clenched around a mother's instinct.
>
> **Coach Daniels:** Caught between duty and the scoreboard.

None of them could know what had just begun.

Not a touchdown. Not a mistake.

A tally. Two hits. Out of 25,000.

Brett's Hidden Record

> **Total Hits (Games + Practices):** 1,275
>
> **Unknown Concussions (Not Reported):** 2 (Suspected)
>
> **Known / Reported Concussions:** 1

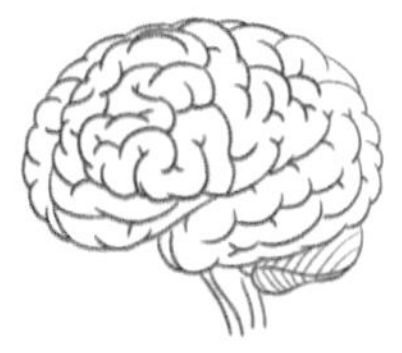

Chapter 2
Tough It Out Culture

Brett

The morning light slanted through the kitchen blinds, stripes of sun and shadow cutting across the table. Brett sat hunched over his cereal, spoon barely moving. His skull throbbed like a slow drumbeat behind his eyes, but he forced a smirk when Braxton, his little brother, burst into the room, voice already at full volume.

"Did it hurt when you hit that guy? You looked like a beast!"

Brett chuckled, but his stomach clenched.

Don't let them see. That was the rule. The first rule. Always.

He'd grown up hearing about his dad playing through broken fingers, cracked ribs, bruises so deep they looked like oil slicks under the skin. Compared to that, what was a headache?

Angela's hand reached across the table, light but searching. She touched his wrist, eyes narrowing.

"You okay?"

Brett flinched, pulling back. "I'm fine, Mom. Just tired."

Tired. The easiest lie.

If she pushed, if she caught on, if word got back to Coach... he could lose everything. His starting spot. His future. His name on that scholarship list.

He swallowed hard, along with another spoonful of cereal, and pulled the armor back over his face.

Tough. Unshakable. Invincible.

Just like he was supposed to be.

The Parentals

Angela stirred cream into her coffee, eyes flicking to Brett like clockwork. Her mind played the replay in a loop. She saw his stumble on the field, the half-second delay, and the way it looked like a shadow was wearing her son's body.

She should say something. Push for a doctor. Rest. Anything, but Marcus's voice cut through her hesitation.

"He's fine, Ange. You worry too much. It's football, he's built for it. I played through worse every Saturday."

Angela sighed. He was right about one thing: she hadn't lived it the way Marcus had. He carried his old injuries like badges of honor. To him, toughness was simply part of the game.

At the end of the table, their ten-year-old twins sat shoulder to shoulder, cereal bowls clinking.

Braxton and Bridgette went to the same school, shared the same birthday, and were almost never apart. But that was where the similarities ended.

Braxton adored his big brother with wide-eyed hero worship. To him, Brett was a superhero in cleats. Every hit he took made him look tougher. Every game was proof that Brett was invincible. If Brett could handle it, football couldn't be dangerous. Brett was built for it. Brett was a beast.

Bridgette didn't buy it. She was smart, unfiltered, and usually right, something that made both her teachers and her parents tread carefully. She loved her brothers, but she would not turn away from the truth. And while Braxton watched Brett with awe, Bridgette watched him with a raised eyebrow. She paid attention to the things others missed. And she had thoughts.

Just then, she leaned across the table, sass sharp in her voice. "Mom's right. Brett looked dizzy last night. If I was Coach, I would've pulled him."

Angela felt a flicker of validation.

Marcus shook his head, hiding a grin. "See? That's what's wrong with football today. Everybody wants to pull kids out for nothing. Back in my day, we shook it off and got back in the game."

Angela's eyes darkened. *And how many hits like that did you take? How many scars are hiding under that pride?*

Coach Daniels

Coach Daniels sat in his office, back stiff against the creaky leather chair, replaying the film from Friday night on his laptop. He quickly tapped the space bar, the screen froze right when Brett stumbled. Daniels leaned forward onto the desk before tapping the space bar again to resume the play and closely watch the way Brett's body drifted half a beat behind the rest of the play.

The pen in his hand tapped like a metronome.

By the book, he knew what this meant: check the kid, pull him if symptoms show. But this was Brett. Their starter. The one with colleges watching. Pulling him now meant shaking momentum. Losing ground. Drawing fire from the athletic director, the boosters, and the town.

He muttered under his breath, "It's just a ding. He'll shake it off and be fine."

But memory scratched at the edges.

Last year's running back had that same stumble. And that same smile that didn't quite reach the eyes.

Until the collapse. Until it was too late.

Daniels shut the laptop with a snap and pushed the thought away like it hadn't crawled into his gut.

The season was too important for what-ifs.

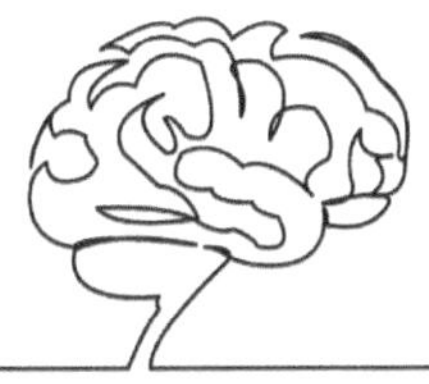

Myths vs. Facts

"It's just a ding."
Even one concussion can alter brain function. Multiple "dings" add up, fast.

"If you don't pass out, it's not serious."
Less than 10% of concussions involve unconsciousness.

"Shaking it off makes you tougher."
It actually makes you more vulnerable to long-term damage.

"A good night's sleep will fix it."
Many symptoms worsen or emerge hours or days later.

These myths don't protect athletes, they protect the silence. And silence is deadly.

Closing Reflection

Three voices, three corners of the same triangle:

Brett: Swallowing his symptoms with cereal and fear.

The Parentals: Split between Marcus' pride and Angela's gnawing instinct.

Coach Daniels: Staring at the film and choosing the scoreboard over the signs.

This was the culture Brett lived in.
Where silence was strength. Pain was currency.
And toughness… was slowly stealing his future.

Brett's Hidden Record

Total Hits (Games + Practices): 1,310

Unknown Concussions (Not Reported): 5 (Suspected)

Known / Reported Concussions: 1

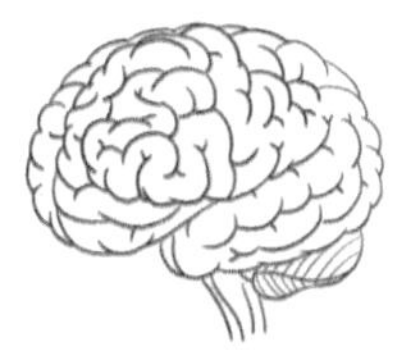

Chapter 3
Practice Makes Pressure

Brett

Tuesday's practice throbbed like another game day, but worse. Brett hadn't felt right since that hit last Friday. The August sun beat down with a vengeance, heat bouncing off the turf in waves that made the field shimmer. Brett squinted through the glare as the whistle split the air.

His helmet already felt too tight.
Like his skull was swelling inside it.

"Line it up again!" Coach Daniels barked.

Brett dropped into his stance, heartbeat hammering in his chest. No breaks. No mercy. Practice wasn't where you coasted. Practice was where you earned your name. And with scouts watching games as well as film, *every snap mattered.*

One misstep and the dream, *his* dream, could crack open and disappear.

The next hit came fast. Helmet to shoulder pad. The jolt exploded through his skull. A familiar high-pitched ringing filled his ears like a swarm of bees trapped in a jar.

His knees dipped. Legs wobbled. But he stayed upright, clenching his jaw against the pain.

Don't let them see. Don't give Coach a reason to doubt me.

Again. And again.

The drills blurred into each other, collisions without names. Hits without count.

All he knew was the rule: *Be perfect. Or lose everything.*

The Parentals

Angela dreaded practice days even more than game days. There were no crowds or camera crews, only brutal repetition hidden from view. And Brett came home looking like he'd fought a war.

Soaked in sweat. Shoulders slumped. Eyes distant.

He sat at the kitchen table too long, elbows on the wood, fingers pressed against his temples like they were holding something inside his head.

"You okay?" she asked gently.

"I'm fine," Brett muttered, lips tugging into a practiced smile.

Marcus clapped him on the back with pride. "That's how you earn it. Practices are where scholarships are won. You can't take plays off."

Angela shook her head. "But at what cost? He's a kid, Marcus. Not a machine."

Marcus barely blinked. "This is the grind. He knows it. I knew it when I was his age. If he wants that scholarship, this is what it takes."

From the hallway, Bridgette's voice sliced through the moment: "Or maybe it just takes brains. Not everyone needs football to go to college."

Braxton, sprawled on the floor with a football in his lap, chimed in without missing a beat: "Yeah, but Brett's gonna make it. He's unstoppable."

Angela's heart ached.

To Bridgette, Brett looked breakable.

To Braxton, he looked bulletproof.

And somewhere between their two truths, the real one was being lost.

Coach Daniels

Daniels stood at the edge of the field, whistle tight in his fist, eyes scanning his players like chess pieces in motion. The sun blazed down. Like always, the turf shimmered with heat. And the sound of helmet on helmet rang like war drums.

They were pushing. Good. That's what it took.

Some critics said they were too hard on these kids. That contact should be limited. That practice should be safer.

Daniels had heard it all before. But he didn't believe in safe toughness. You couldn't theory your way into grit. You earned it in collisions.

Still, his eyes tracked Brett.

The kid stumbled between drills. Not big. Just a half-step, like his body wasn't quite syncing with his mind.

Daniels frowned.

He's tougher than most, Daniels told himself, forcing the doubt back down. *Kid's carrying a lot. Scouts. Family. Pressure. Let him fight through it.*

"Shake it off, Brett! Line up again!"

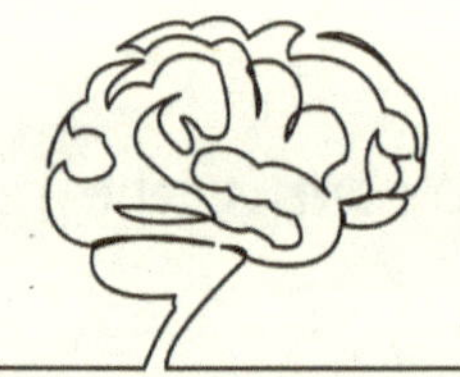

Concussion by the Numbers

3.8 million: Estimated sports-related concussions in the U.S. each year

50%: Athletes who don't report their concussion symptoms

1 in 5: High school athletes who will suffer a second concussion in the same season

15–24 years: The most at-risk age group

30%: Concussions worsen when athletes return to play too soon

The numbers show what the culture hides: concussions are common, underreported, and far more dangerous when ignored.

Time Out: Reflection

Three forces drove the pressure that built on Brett's shoulders:

Brett: Pushing through brutal drills while his head pounded and the dream pulled further out of reach.

The Parentals: Marcus glorifying the grind, Angela watching her son unravel.

Coach Daniels: Who saw the signs but clung to toughness as the only answer.

The cracks were there, visible if you knew where to look.

But in a world that worshipped toughness, cracks were ignored.

Brett's Hidden Record

Total Hits (Games + Practices): 1,340

Unknown Concussions (Not Reported): 6 (Suspected)

Known / Reported Concussions: 1

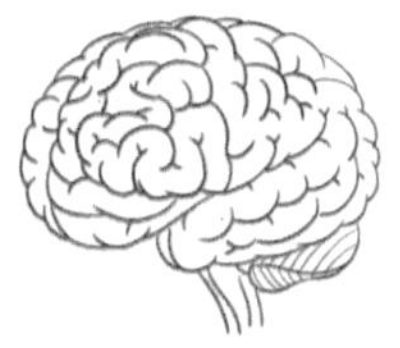

Second Quarter
The Big Stage

Kickoff

High school ended in a blur of caps, gowns, and Friday night memories that the whole town swore they'd never forget. When Brett walked across the graduation stage, his name echoed through the auditorium like a hometown victory chant. To them, he was proof that small-town grit could lead to something greater.

The scholarship letter from Jefferson Commonwealth University was already framed above the fireplace. Jefferson wasn't just any school. Its stadium, nicknamed The Iron Bowl, rose in Virginia like a monument to football. Playing there had been Brett's dream since he was a little kid watching his father's old game tapes. Now it was real.

Angela cried when he signed the papers. Marcus gripped his son's hand with the quiet pride of a man reliving his own glory days. Bridgette rolled her eyes and called dibs on his room. Braxton told anyone who'd listen that his brother was a JC Cougar and about to play for the best team in the country.

But for Brett, the celebration carried a sharper edge. The hits would be faster now. The players bigger. The risks heavier. Every snap was a test and every mistake was a threat to the scholarship that held his family's hopes.

The whistle blew again. The First Quarter was over. Now Brett stepped into the Second, The Big Stage. The game was faster now and the stakes were higher.

Enter Coach Reynolds

On the first day of training camp, Brett met Coach Reynolds, the head coach at Jefferson. He was tall, barrel-chested, and spoke with a voice that seemed to shake the turf itself. His reputation was already legendary, demanding, relentless and impossible to please.

"Welcome to college ball," Reynolds said, his voice booming. "If you thought high school was tough, forget it. This is faster, harder and meaner. You're not boys anymore. You're warriors. And warriors don't complain about bruises."

Brett's stomach clenched.

He means me. He's watching. I can't stumble. I can't slip. If I do, my scholarship and my future are gone.

The voice inside his helmet came rushing back, only louder now.

Don't let them see. Don't let them think you're weak. Not here. Not now.

Coach Daniels had been the voice of high school grit. Now Coach Reynolds was the voice of college survival. Brett stood between both echoes, still clinging to the belief that toughness was the only way through.

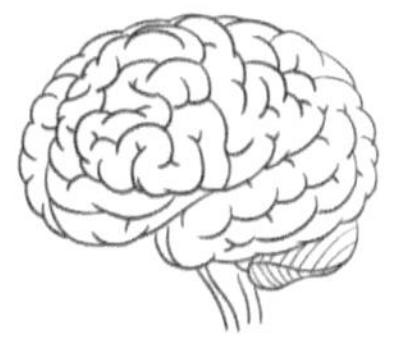

Chapter 4
The Big Stage

Brett

The stadium towered around him, louder and brighter than anything Brett had ever known. The lights stretched into the sky, a second sun over a sea of strangers. The first time he stepped onto the turf in his college uniform, his chest tightened.

Scholarships weren't guaranteed. Playing time wasn't promised. Every snap was a test. Every mistake was a threat.

The quarterback's voice thundered through the huddle.

"Ace left, 42 zone, on one. Ready—break!"

The ball snapped. Brett surged forward.

The lineman across from him was faster. Stronger. He hit like a wrecking ball. Brett's helmet snapped back. His teeth crashed against the mouthguard. His balance teetered as he staggered, half a step behind the play.

He caught himself, barely, and pushed forward.

The speed left no room for thinking. High school hits had felt like car crashes. These felt like pileups.

Handle it. You have to handle it. If you don't, the scholarship is gone. The future is gone.

His vision cleared just as the next play was called.

And the next hit.

The Parentals

Angela gripped the stadium railing so tight, her knuckles turned white. The roar of the crowd pulsed around her, but all she saw was Brett. He appeared smaller now, swallowed in a storm of bigger, older, faster men.

"Look at him out there," Marcus said, swelling with pride. "He's holding his own."

Angela's eyes narrowed. "You don't see how hard those hits are? This isn't high school anymore. These aren't boys. They're grown men."

Marcus crossed his arms. "That's the next level. He's earning it."

Bridgette, now eleven but just as razor-sharp, leaned over with a smirk. "Or breaking himself for it."

Beside her, Braxton beamed, eyes locked on the field like he was watching a superhero. "That's my brother. He's unstoppable."

Angela's heart twisted.

To Marcus, this was progress.

To Bridgette, it was danger wrapped in a uniform.

To Braxton, it was a dream unfolding in real time.

But to her, it looked like her son was being pulled deeper into something none of them could slow down.

I'm the only one who sees what's really happening. Aren't I?

Coach Reynolds

Coach Reynolds stood stone-faced on the sideline, arms folded. His voice rolled across the field like distant thunder. His presence alone seemed to command the stadium.

"This is college ball," he'd told the rookies. "It's faster. It's harder. It's unforgiving. If you can't handle it, the bench is waiting. Warriors don't complain."

Now he watched Brett from across the field. The kid was tough. Disciplined. Determined to earn his place. Everything Reynolds respected.

But when Brett took a hit and took too long getting up, the coach's jaw tightened.

He didn't ask. Didn't pause. Just barked.

"Keep driving, Taylor. Don't you dare slow down!"

Still, a thought crept in.

How long can he take these hits before they take something from him?

Reynolds shoved it down. There was no room for doubt.

In this world, grit earned scholarships. And silence kept you in the game.

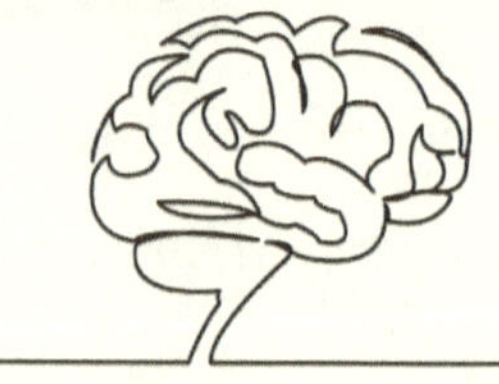

Why Speed and Force Increase Traumatic Brain Injuries (TBI) Risk

Faster game, harder impacts. College athletes move faster and hit harder, increasing the severity of every collision.

Physics of hits. Force = mass X acceleration. Bigger, faster players mean more impact energy driven into the brain.

Invisible toll. Even when athletes don't show obvious signs of injury, the brain still absorbs the force of rapid movement and twisting inside the skull. Over time, that stress can accumulate and cause damage.

As the game speeds up,
so does the danger. Progress on the field comes
at a cost inside the skull.

TIME OUT: Reflection

Three perspectives stood at the edge of Brett's new reality:

> **Brett:** Grinding through hits that came faster and landed harder, clinging to his scholarship.
>
> **The Parentals:** Marcus proud, Angela afraid, Bridgette skeptical, Braxton in awe.
>
> **Coach Reynolds:** Watching closely, but choosing silence over caution.

The stage was bigger now. The players stronger. The pressure heavier.

But one truth hadn't changed since the first quarter.

Every hit still counted.

Brett's Hidden Record

> **Total Hits (Games + Practices):** 1,670
>
> **Unknown Concussions (Not Reported):** 10 (Suspected)
>
> **Known / Reported Concussions:** 1

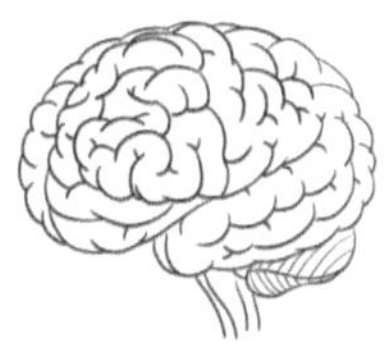

Chapter 5
The Invisible Ledger

Brett

By midseason, Brett's body moved on autopilot. His legs ran the drills. His hands fought through blocks. But his mind…his mind lagged behind.

In practice, the quarterback shouted a play.

"Trips right, 36 power, X slant!"

Brett froze.

Just a second. Just long enough for his chest to tighten.

What did he just say?

He guessed his spot in the formation and hoped no one noticed.

But it didn't stop on the field.

In the locker room, small things slipped.

He'd forget where he left his cleats.

Mix up lift days.

Stumble on the name of a teammate he'd met three times.

His head throbbed constantly now. A steady, dull ache that clung to him from sunrise to sunset. But he chalked it up to stress.

What scared him more were the mood swings. One minute he was laughing on FaceTime with Braxton, the next he snapped at Bridgette for teasing him about forgetting her birthday call.

His own voice startled him. It sounded too sharp. Too fast. Like someone else's.

And off the field, it showed up in other ways.

College had promised everything, bigger stadiums, louder crowds, and more attention. Especially from girls. Brett had always been smooth when it came to the ladies. High school had been easy.

But now? Between team workouts, film, practices, classes, study hall, and games, Brett barely had time to breathe. He wanted to go out, to be seen, and to just feel normal. But the nights slipped away. The invitations piled up. And dating became a disaster.

Brett started mixing up names. Forgetting who he'd promised to call. He was showing up late, or not at all. And his temper flared when he was called out for it.

It wasn't him. But admitting that felt like opening a door he couldn't close.

So, he shut it instead.

I'm too busy. No dating during football season.

That was the line. Easy. Clean. Focused.

It wasn't the truth.

But it kept people from looking too closely.

You can't admit this.

You can't let it slip.

They'll think you're weak and take it all away.

So, Brett stayed quiet.

Don't let them see. Don't give anyone a reason to doubt you.

The Parentals

Even over the phone, Angela heard it.

The way Brett's voice clipped the ends of his sentences. How it drifted when she asked about classes. How it snapped when she pushed too hard.

"You sound tired," she said gently.

"I'm fine, Mom. Just practice."

But when she hung up, her gut didn't settle.

She turned to Marcus in the kitchen. "He's forgetting things and he snapped at me again. I am telling you, honey, something's not right."

Marcus shook his head. "He's adjusting. College ball is pressure. He'll come through."

Bridgette, sat at the table with a math workbook open, barely looked up.

"He's not fine. He's meaner now. Don't you hear it?"

Braxton yelled from the living room while tossing up a football.

"He's just focused. He's got to be. This is the big leagues."

Angela sighed. To Bridgette, Brett was changing in ways no one wanted to see. To Braxton, he was just becoming the hero he always believed in. To Marcus, it was all part of the grind.

But to her, it felt like something invisible was stealing pieces of her son. And nobody else seemed to be noticing.

Coach Reynolds

Coach Reynolds prided himself on reading his players' body language, effort, and attitude. But with Brett, he saw what he wanted to see.

The kind of kid who pushed through pain and who made teams win.

But even he couldn't ignore the signs.

A missed assignment. A half-step delay on the snap. A flash of temper during a rep.

The trainer mentioned it once. "Coach, Taylor says he's foggy and he's been coming in with headaches."

Reynolds waved it off. "Everyone's banged up this time of year. Tape him. Ice him. Get him ready."

He didn't believe in pulling starters for headaches. That wasn't how the game worked. Not here.

Still, deep down, a voice whispered something he didn't want to hear.

It's not just bruises anymore.

Each hit added to a debt nobody tracked. Not on paper or in the playbook.

But the toll was real.

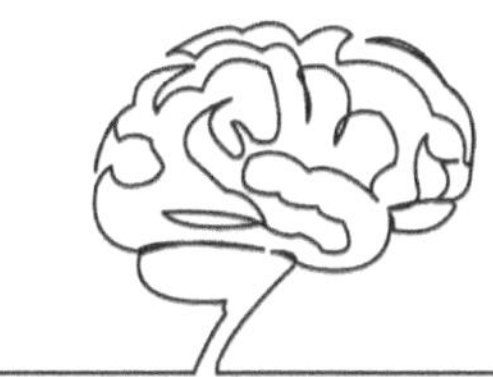

Dr. Omalu and the 25,000 Collisions

Dr. Bennet Omalu, a Nigerian-born forensic pathologist, was the first to discover Chronic Traumatic Encephalopathy (CTE) in the brain of former NFL player Mike Webster.

When he examined Webster's brain, he described it as being in the condition of a man who had survived 25,000 car crashes.

Over time, these "invisible hits" accumulated, breaking the brain from the inside out.

Every collision left its mark, even the ones that didn't cause a concussion.

The brain recorded each impact, whether or not the body showed signs.

The Invisible Ledger: It's not just the big knockouts, it's the thousands of smaller hits that adds up over time.

Closing Reflection

Four perspectives pointed to what no one wanted to name:

Brett: Slipping deeper into fog through flashes of anger and silence.

The Parentals: Watching from a distance, Angela notices a change and Marcus dismisses it.

The Siblings: Bridgette calling it out and Braxton refusing to believe it.

Coach Reynolds: Ignoring the signs while trusting toughness over truth.

The scoreboard measured wins.
But Brett's brain was keeping a tally of its own.
And no one was ready to read the ledger.

Brett's Hidden Record

Total Hits (Games + Practices): 1,900

Unknown Concussions (Not Reported): 12 (Suspected)

Known / Reported Concussions: 1

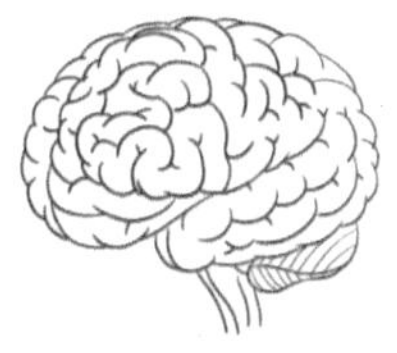

Chapter 6
The Hit That Lingers

Brett

The play unfolded in a blur.

Brett exploded off the line, helmet colliding with a defender's shoulder. The crack tore through his skull like a bolt of lightning. For a moment, he stayed upright, feet moving on instinct.

Then the world tilted.

The turf rushed up fast.

He heard the crowd gasp as his body hit the ground, but inside his head there was only silence. There was no roar or sound of whistles. The silence was thick and heavy.

When his eyes blinked open, the stadium lights stabbed through like knives. He squinted, disoriented, trying to push himself up. His legs trembled and refused to cooperate.

Trainers swarmed, he felt hands firm on his shoulders.

"Stay down, Brett. Stay still."

No. No. No.

Don't let them see me weak. Don't let them think I'm broken.

He forced a shaky grin as they helped him toward the sideline. "I'm fine. Just slipped," he muttered, even as his stomach churned and his vision blurred.

The word protocol floated around him. It felt hollow, like a checklist. Just another thing to get through.

He already knew how this went.

They would hold him out and ask a few questions. Then they would clear him and he'd be back in the game.

The Parentals

Angela's heart stopped the moment Brett went down.

She grabbed Marcus's arm so hard he hissed. "Marcus! Marcus, did you see that? He's hurt. He went down hard."

Marcus leaned forward, jaw tight. "He'll be fine. The trainers are with him."

But Angela wasn't listening anymore.

She saw the way Brett struggled to stand. The way his legs wobbled like they didn't belong to him and the way his smile didn't reach his eyes.

"That's not fine," she said, her voice rising. "That's not fine!"

Bridgette, a few rows down, turned toward them, her face flushed. "He doesn't even know where he is," she said flatly.

"You still think this is nothing?"

Braxton's voice floated over, bright and certain. "He's just shaking it off like he always does. He'll be back, trust me"

Angela snapped.

"THAT'S ENOUGH," she exclaimed stomping her foot into the floor of the bleachers.

Marcus turned, startled. "Angela, calm down."

"NO," she demanded, now standing, her hands were shaking. "I am done calming down."

Heads turned. She didn't care.

"I told you something was wrong," she said, her voice cracking and climbing at the same time. "I told you after high school. I told you after practice. I told you when he started forgetting things. And every time you told me I was worrying too much."

Marcus opened his mouth. She didn't let him speak.

"I stood by you. I trusted you. I told myself you knew the game better than I did. Her voice broke.

"And look where that got us."

Marcus stared at the field, silent now.

"That is our son out there," she said, pointing. "Our baby. And I knew. I knew something wasn't right. And I let you talk me out of it."

Her anger turned inward, sharp and sudden.

"I should have taken him to a doctor. I should have demanded answers. I should have listened to myself instead of being afraid of being the difficult one."

Tears spilled over, hot and furious.

"This is on you," she said, voice shaking. "But it's on me too."

Angela stood there, breath unsteady, watching trainers guide her son away.

Moments later, the crowd roared as the game resumed, as if nothing ever happened.

Coach Reynolds

From the sideline, Coach Reynolds kept his face unreadable.

Inside, his stomach twisted.

A star player going down mid-game was every coach's nightmare.

The trainer leaned in "We're Starting concussion protocol. He's disoriented."

Reynolds exhaled sharply, then barked "Run the checklist! Do your job and don't drag this out."

He told himself it was practical, not cruel. Football was violent and players got hit. They got cleared and went back in.

That was all part of the game.

Still, as he watched Brett sway, his eyes looked glassy, and doubt crept in.

How many more times can a kid get up like that before he doesn't?

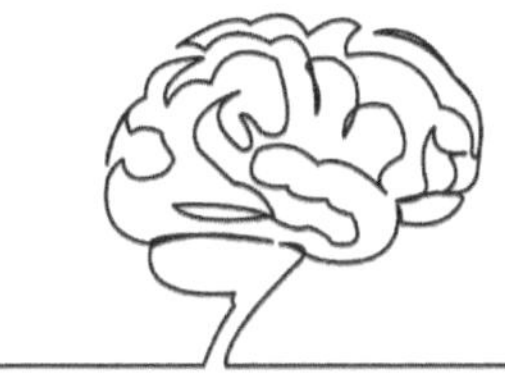

Persistent Post-Concussion Syndrome (PPCS)

Persistent post-concussive symptoms (PPCS) occur when symptoms last longer than expected, typically beyond four weeks in youth or three months in adults.

Symptoms may include:

- Persistent headaches or migraines
- Dizziness and balance problems
- Sensitivity to light and sound
- Memory and concentration difficulties
- Mood swings, anxiety, or depression
- Sleep disturbances

Many athletes are told they'll bounce back in a week or two. For those with PPCS, the hit lingers far beyond the field, affecting school, relationships, and daily life.

Closing Reflection

Three perspectives marked the night Brett collapsed:

Brett: Desperate to minimize his symptoms and terrified of being labeled fragile.

The Parentals: no longer divided quietly. Marcus clinging to toughness. Angela done ignoring her instincts.

Coach Reynolds: Staring at the cost of a protocol built on silence.

The crowd moved on.

The game continued.

But this hit did not fade.

It lingered.

And so did the truth Angela could no longer ignore.

Brett's Hidden Record

Total Hits (Games + Practices): 2,150

Unknown Concussions (Not Reported): 13 (Suspected)

Known / Reported Concussions: 1

End of the Second Quarter

The scoreboard told one story: Brett's team was leading at halftime. The crowd cheered, the band played, and the stadium pulsed with energy.

But Brett's body was telling a different story, one marked by the collapse, the fog, and the sharp light piercing his eyes. To Marcus, it looked like grit, while Angela saw a warning she couldn't ignore. Bridgette recognized the danger, Braxton saw something to admire, and Coach Reynolds viewed it as a problem to manage.

The truth was harder than anyone wanted to admit. Brett had been playing through an invisible injury, one the game was never built to recognize.

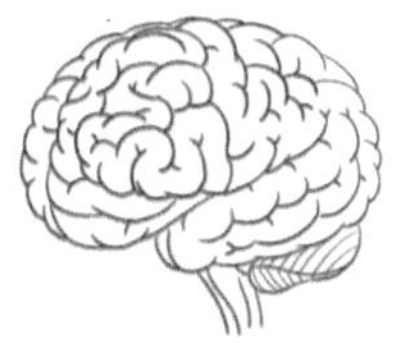

Third Quarter: Breaking Point

Breaking Point

Halftime was supposed to be for adjustments, for rest, for planning the next play. But Brett's halftime was spent contemplating what was to come next.

He had made it through high school glory and the grind of college ball. He had survived brutal practices, hidden concussions, and even collapsing under stadium lights. But now, the cost was catching up. The hits weren't just part of the game anymore, they were part of him.

The Third Quarter would not be about chasing scholarships or earning playing time. It would be about survival. About learning what it meant to live with the consequences.

About the slow, invisible breaking point that football had set in motion.

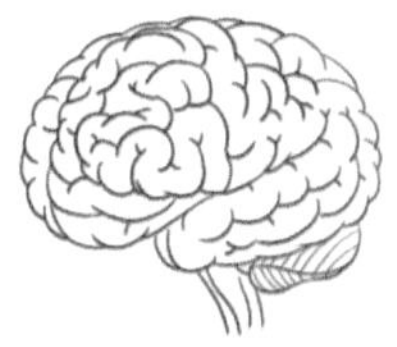

Chapter 7
Silence and Struggle

Brett

It had been weeks since Brett's concussion. But the days blurred together now. Brett woke up groggy, stumbling through classes with a fog that never seemed to lift. The fluorescent lights in lecture halls stabbed his eyes, making it hard to focus on the slides. He squinted, blinking hard, but the words slipped past him.

Assignments piled up. His grades, once steady, began to drop. He snapped at friends over nothing. One moment he was joking around, the next he was slamming his fist against his desk in a rage he couldn't explain, one that boiled up without warning.

Things even felt "off" on the field. Now, Brett hesitated before every snap, and the playbook suddenly felt foreign in his hands. During practices he missed reads he would normally make without thinking, the game was suddenly moving faster than his mind could process.

At night, sleep wouldn't come. When it did, it was restless. He'd wake up drenched in sweat, heart pounding, head throbbing.

The trainers had cleared him, and told him he was "fine."

But nothing about this felt fine. It felt permanent.

And one night, it broke.

Unable to sleep, Brett sat on the edge of his bed, holding his head in his hands as the ache pulsed behind his eyes. His breath caught. His chest tightened. And for the first time in years, Brett cried.

Silent at first. Then harder.

He didn't know what scared him more, the tears or the fact that he didn't understand why they were there.

He didn't feel injured. He felt...lost.

Don't let them see. Don't let them know you're slipping.

But the tears kept coming, warm and steady, streaking down his face as his mind spiraled with a question he didn't know how to answer.

What's happening to me?

He wanted to sleep. God, he wanted to sleep. But nothing worked. Not music. Not deep breathing. Not the blackout curtains he'd put up last week.

So, Brett lay awake, his pillow damp, his hands clenched.

He replayed what he could remember about missed assignments, forgotten plays, and the names that vanished mid-sentence.

And just before sleep finally pulled him under, one thought surfaced through the fog.

I want my mom.

The Parentals

Angela stared at the midterm grades in her email inbox, her stomach twisting.

C's. D's. One class marked incomplete.

Brett had never been a straight-A student, but he'd always tried. Always cared. This wasn't just slipping.

She decided to call him that night.

"Honey, what's going on? These grades...this is not like you."

"I'm just...tired, Mom. College is harder, that's all."

But it wasn't just his words. It was his voice. It was flat, short, and impatient. He didn't ask about the family. He no longer joked. He didn't sound like her Brett.

Angela sat on the couch after the call with the phone in her lap and heart pounding.

Marcus glanced over. "Stay calm, I know you're worried but he'll bounce back like he always does. It's midterms Ange. The boy just needs a break."

Angela shook her head slowly. "He's not just tired. I feel like he's unraveling."

Bridgette didn't even look up from her homework. "Told you."

Angela exhaled hard and closed the laptop.

She had tried to be supportive. To wait it out. To believe Marcus when he said it was normal. But this wasn't normal. And she was done waiting.

Brett would be coming home for the long weekend in a few day. And this time, she wouldn't back down. Not again. She'd sit him down and make him talk. Really talk.

No more pretending.

No more silence.

Coach Reynolds

Coach Reynolds noticed the change on the field. Brett was slower. Sloppier. His eyes looked dull. His temper lit like a fuse during drills.

The trainers shrugged it off. "Headaches with some fatigue, but that's nothing that flags protocol."

Reynolds didn't like excuses. Headaches didn't lose games. Weakness did.

Still... he couldn't shake the unease. Brett had always been sharp. Now, he looked like a kid trying to remember where to go.

"Get your head right, Taylor. We need you focused."

But even as he barked the words, a voice in the back of his mind whispered: *What if he can't?*

Flashback – 11 Years Earlier

Reynold's thought back to his high school coaching days. He hadn't said the name out loud in years.

Conner Snowhill.

Sno, as the players had called him, was the kind of kid who turned heads. He was fast, ferocious, a magnet for scouts. By his senior year, Sno had more D1 offers than anyone Reynolds had ever coached. Bigger schools. Bigger dreams. He was tough in the way only seventeen-year-olds trying to escape their zip code can be.

Reynolds had admired that toughness. Loved it, even.

Just like Brett.

That's what scared him now.

The memories came back in sequence: the concussion two weeks before the state championship, the way Sno had stumbled through drills in the days that followed, saying he was "just a little off." Protocol back then was looser. Loopholes wider. A doctor's note from Sno's parents appeared, and he'd been cleared to play.

So, who was Reynolds to argue?

Everyone wanted it. The team. The town. The stands were packed. Signs waved. "WAY TO GO SNO."

And for the first half, Sno was electric. Running backs bounced off him. The sideline was buzzing.

Then came the hit.

A blindside collision…full speed, helmet to helmet. Sno dropped like a sack of bricks. No movement. No sound.

Reynolds squeezed his eyes shut even now, trying not to see it.

The trainer's voice still rang in his ears. *"We've got a problem."*

Sno was airlifted to the hospital and diagnosed with Second Impact Syndrome.

Coma. Six weeks. Then...nothing. Life support was removed. A funeral held.

After the funeral, Reynolds did his best to shove down memories of Sno.

He never told anyone how many times he'd replayed the choice of taking the note, and sending Sno in, to chase a trophy. Telling himself it was what winners did.

Now, watching Brett move slower, forget plays, and flinch at light...he saw it again.

The same drive.

The same determination.

And possibly at risk of experiencing the same ending.

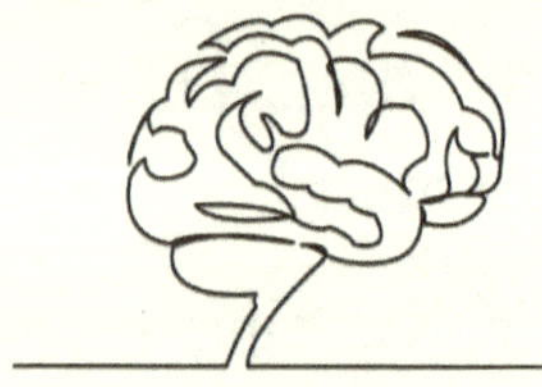

Long-Term Effects of Repeated Brain Trauma

Repeated concussions and sub-concussive hits can cause long-lasting effects, even years after the athlete stops playing.

Cognitive:

Memory loss

Difficulty concentrating

Slowed processing speed

Emotional/Behavioral:

Mood swings

Depression and anxiety

Irritability, aggression

Physical:

Chronic headaches

Sensitivity to light and sound

Sleep disturbances

Second Impact Syndrome (SIS) *is a rare but deadly condition that occurs when a second concussion happens before the first one has fully healed. The brain swells rapidly, often with catastrophic consequences.*

Even young, healthy athletes can suffer fatal outcomes if returned to play too soon.

Closing Reflection

Three perspectives revealed the silent struggle:

Brett: Drowning in fog, rage, and sleepless nights, trying to keep it hidden.

The Parentals: Watching his grades slip and his personality shift. Angela ready to confront what she had tried to ignore.

Coach Reynolds: Seeing the symptoms, still refusing to name the cost.

Brett's Hidden Record

Total Hits (Games + Practices): 2,450

Unknown Concussions (Not Reported): 15 (Suspected)

Known / Reported Concussions: 2

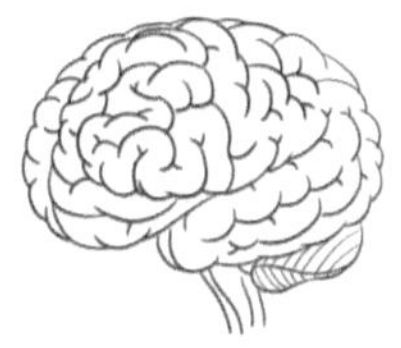

Chapter 8
The Spark of Knowledge

Brett

Brett was home for the long weekend. He sat slumped on the couch, scrolling mindlessly through his phone when Bridgette burst through the door, backpack bouncing against her shoulders. Her eyes were wide and her voice spilled out like a dam had broken.

"Brett! You're not gonna believe what I learned today! They had this thing at school called "Brain Talk Day" and Dr. Kelli was there! She taught us all about this egg thing."

Brett frowned. "Egg thing?"

"Yeah. She said your brain is like the raw yolk inside an eggshell. If you shake it around, even if the shell doesn't break, the yolk inside still gets messed up. That's what happens in your head when you take hits on the football field. Even if you wear a helmet and look fine on the outside, the inside can still be scrambled."

Brett blinked. The analogy hit harder than he expected. It felt too real.

Bridgette's tone softened. "Brett…you're so different now… you forget stuff. You snap at Brax and me all the time. And you're even mean to Mommy sometimes. Annnnnnd you always have a headache. That's what Dr. Kelli talked about. She said those are signs."

He tried to laugh it off, but the sound came out hollow. "You're ten, Bridge. You don't know what you're talking about."

But Bridgette wasn't done. She threw her hands on her tiny hips, eyes fiery. "First of all, I'm eleven now, remember? And second, prove me wrong. Listen to her podcast. It's called *Kandid Konversations with Dr. Kelli*. She had a football player's mom on there. He was your age when his symptoms started, and he had the same problems as you. Like your headaches, forgetting things and being a big meany! He didn't think it was a big deal either."

Brett swallowed hard, unease creeping into his chest. "And?" he asked.

Her voice dropped, her sass replaced with something heavier. "He died! By suicide..and his mom said it was CTE."

As she turned to leave the room, Brett heard her say, "Nobody ever listens to me…what do I know…I am just an eleven year old."

Bridgette's words slammed into Brett like a hit he couldn't brace for.

He'd heard about CTE before and even read headlines about NFL players. His teammates often made jokes about it in the locker room. "Better enjoy the game now before we all get

CTE," the guys used to laugh after brutal practices. Nobody ever thought it could happen to them. It was something that happened to the old pros, the retired legends but not to kids and not to players his age.

Now, hearing Bridgette's words, it didn't feel like a joke anymore. And for the first time, Brett felt afraid.

The room went quiet. Then, Brett felt that familiar tightening in his chest. He wanted to say that Bridgette was being dramatic and that he wasn't going out like that.

But then the vulnerability surfaced beneath it all…the fear he'd shoved down for months.

Warm tears began to fall.

Warriors don't feel. Don't let them see. Don't let them know you're slipping, he thought as the tears streamed down his cheeks.

He realized he had no clue what was happening to him or how much more he could take.

The Parentals

That night, after putting the twins to bed, Angela sat alone at the kitchen table with her laptop open. She searched the podcast Bridgette had mentioned at dinner, *Kandid Konversations with Dr. Kelli.*

She found it, Season Two, Episode Three: "A Mother's Story: Football, CTE, and the Son I Lost."

Angela took a slow breath and pressed play.

Halfway through the episode, she heard the mother's voice crack with grief. Every word was soaked in pain. She described noticing changes in her happy, charismatic child. Angela listened the familiar symptoms: headaches, memory troubles, and mood swings. These were echoes of everything Angela had been afraid to name.

As the episode concluded, the mom's emotion filled message to parents cut Angela the deepest:

> Parents, stay in your kids' faces. Don't give up on your kids. If your gut tells you that something is wrong, follow your gut—listen to your gut. Don't make the same mistake I did by explaining the signs away.
>
> It's one of the most powerful tools that we have—our own bodies—and listening to our own body and the messages it sends us. If you're blessed enough to still have your kid alive, do whatever it takes to get through to them. Because nothing is worth it. Not money, not houses, not cars. I'd give anything to get my baby back.

Angela wiped tears from her cheeks. Her mind flashed to Marcus dismissing her worries, to Braxton's hero worship, and to Bridgette's fierce honesty.

Most of all, she thought of Brett. Her baby was still here and still alive but he was still slipping away.

It was time for a "Kandid Konversation" of her own. And this time she would not back down.

The Confrontation

The next night, Brett sat at the kitchen table, hunched over a plate of leftovers. Fork in hand, hoodie pulled up halfway, his eyes looked hollow under the dim light. He wasn't really tasting the food, just chewing through the silence.

Angela stepped into the kitchen, her movements deliberate. Behind her came Marcus, tall, broad-shouldered, silent. He didn't speak, but his presence filled the room like a warning.

Brett looked up, sensing something was off.

Angela didn't waste time. "We need to talk."

He sighed. "About what now?"

"Your grades," she said with a voice steady. "We need to talk about your moods and these headaches that you have all the time. Bridgette's worried and I'm worried, too."

He rolled his eyes. "So this is an ambush, got it!"

Angela firmly pushed back. "Don't be disrespectful, this is not an ambush, Brett. It's your life. I listened to that podcast. You sound just like what that boy's mom described: tired, angry, and confused."

Marcus still hadn't spoken. He leaned against the fridge, arms folded and watching.

Brett shoved his fork into the plate. "You've been listening to *Bridgette* and some woman crying on a podcast who doesn't even know me? I'm fine!"

Angela didn't flinch. "You're not. And deep down, you know it."

Brett's body tensed. The pressure inside him built until it had nowhere else to go. With a sudden, violent motion, he slammed his tightly closed fist onto the table, BOOM! The sound echoed through the kitchen. The plate rattled, fork jumped. A startled Angela gasped and clutched her chest.

He stood abruptly, chair scraping across the floor. His chest rose and fell fast.

His eyes, once full of quiet restrain, now blazed with something sharper, something angrier. He pointed at her, voice raw.

He exploded, *"Stop treating me like I'm broken! I'm not broken, so why don't you just get off my damn back!"*

Marcus lunged forward.

In one swift move, he grabbed Brett by the collar and yanked him away from Angela. The motion was forceful and primal.

"Don't you ever speak to your mother like that again," Marcus growled, low and deadly.

His grip tightened.

Angela's eyes went wide. *"Marcus, stop! Don't hurt him! He's not himself!"*

Marcus' face, burning with rage, began to shift. Slowly, the spell broke. He blinked and looked down…this wasn't a disrespectful young man. This was his son…his boy.

He let go.

Brett staggered backwards, his eyes still filled with rage. In a flash, he turned to leave. Angela asked, "Where are you going?"

Brett barked back, "I'm going for a walk." She tried to go after him but before she could take a step, Marcus' massive arm blocked her. When they locked eyes, he whispered, "Let him go."

Angela wiped the tears from her cheeks. The kitchen felt heavy the air was thick with what almost happened.

In the living room, Bridgette lay still on the couch. Her eyes were shut tight as she pretended to be sleeping, but she'd heard it all. She'd been waiting for this moment. Her mother's voice sliced through the tension one last time, sharp and quiet:

"Keep it down…you'll wake up Bridgette."

Brigette, the Silent Witness

Braxton was at a sleepover and missed it.

But Bridgette lay curled up on the couch in the living room, face toward the cushions, eyes shut tight. She'd heard her mom's warning, *"Keep it down…you'll wake up Bridgette."* But she wasn't asleep, not even close.

She knew that if her mom caught her awake, she'd be sent upstairs, out of earshot.

And Bridgette wasn't about to miss this.

This was the moment she'd sensed building, ever since the midterms, the podcasts and the parentals' quiet talks behind closed doors. She had waited for the explosion. For the truth to finally hit the air like a spark in dry grass.

With her eyes squeezed closed he just listened, holding her breath, her small body still as a statue, smiling faintly to herself.

Finally, she thought. *They're talking about it.*

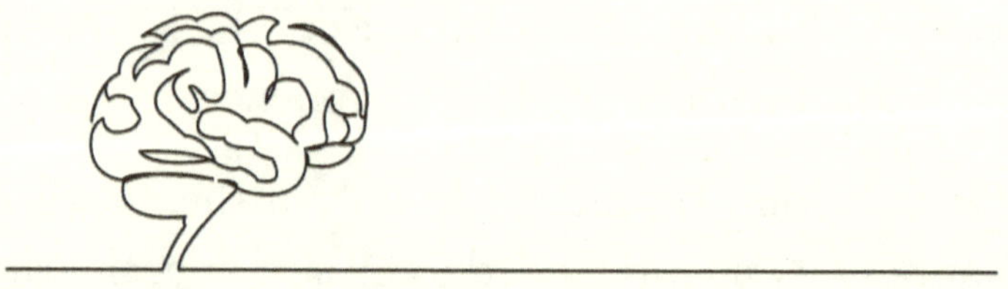

Why Education and Advocacy Matter

Concussions are often called the "invisible injury." Without education, symptoms are dismissed, and athletes keep playing through dangerous hits.

Why education matters:

- Helps families recognize the warning signs
- Gives athletes language to describe their symptoms
- Prevents tragedies by breaking the cycle of silence

Why advocacy matters:

- Challenges cultural myths like "tough it out"
- Pushes schools, teams, and organizations to adopt safer policies
- Provides hope to families who feel powerless

Awareness changes outcomes.
A "Kandid Konversation" shared in a classroom, a podcast, or at the dinner table, can be the spark that saves a life.

Closing Reflection

Three voices carried the spark:

Brett: Shaken by Bridgette's words and the haunting podcast story that mirrored his own.

Angela: Listening to a grieving mother's call to action and finding the courage to confront and her protect her son.

Bridgette: Unapologetically raising awareness for Brett about what his symptoms could really mean.

Brett's Hidden Record

Total Hits (Games + Practices): 2,750

Unknown Concussions (Not Reported): 17 (Suspected)

Known / Reported Concussions: 2

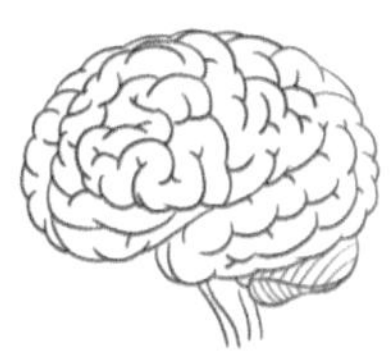

Chapter 9
The Hardest Choice

Brett

By sophomore year, Brett had read more medical journals and athlete memoirs than he ever thought possible. Late nights once spent watching film were now devoted to scrolling through research on CTE, concussion, and post-concussion syndrome. His search history looked nothing like his teammates'.

What started with Bridgette's blunt warning had grown into an obsession. He listened to every episode of *Kandid Konversations with Dr. Kelli*. Retired athletes spoke about memory lapses, mood swings, and the hollow silence after their careers ended. Some shared hope and stories of rebuilding a life outside of sport. Others shared grief.

The more Brett listened, the more unsettled he became. Each symptom they described was his own. Headaches that lingered. Brain fog in class. Mood swings that scared him. Difficulty reading under fluorescent lights. It all sounded too familiar and hit too close to home.

For weeks, he carried the weight of a decision he didn't want to face. Walking away felt like failure. Failure to his team and to Coach Reynolds, who had pushed him hard. To his parents, who had trained him to never give up. To Braxton, who idolized him. To Bridgette, who always expected him to be strong.

But the truth was undeniable. "You only get one brain," Brett whispered to himself one night, staring at his reflection in the dorm bathroom mirror. For the past seven years, he had been taking hit after hit, ignoring every warning sign. He had been gambling with his future, and the odds were turning against him.

Brett thought about the retired players who talked about dementia in their twenties and thirties, about lives cut short by CTE. He thought about the grieving mother's voice on Dr. Kelli's podcast: *"If you're blessed enough to still have your kid alive, do whatever it takes to get through to them."*

Brett realized the bravest thing he could do wasn't stepping back onto the field. It was stepping away from it.

The Parentals

The day Brett told his family, the room was heavy with silence. Angela reached for his hand immediately. Marcus folded his arms, staring at his son as if he'd spoken a foreign language.

"I've been doing research," Brett said carefully. "I can't ignore the symptoms anymore. The headaches and the mood swings… the memory stuff, it all lines up with CTE."

Angela's eyes filled with tears. She thought back to the podcast episode, to the mother's tearful plea. "I'm so proud of you," she whispered. "This is the hardest choice, but it's the right one."

Marcus shook his head. "You're throwing it all away, son. You've worked your whole life for this."

Brett met his father's eyes, his voice steady. "No, Dad. I've worked my whole life for a future and I want to live long enough to actually have one."

In that moment, Angela squeezed his hand tighter. Bridgette leaned against the wall, smirking just slightly as if to say *finally*. Braxton's eyes welled, torn between disappointment and admiration.

Coach Reynolds

Brett stood in Coach Reynolds's office, his helmet resting on the desk like an artifact.

"I'm stepping away, Coach," Brett said, his voice trembling.

Reynolds leaned back in his office chair, arms crossed, staring at the helmet. For a moment, he said nothing. He thought of Sno and remembered the letter from his parents, the signatures on the waiver, Sno's collapse and the deafening silence in the hospital room.

Part of him had feared this moment would come too late.

"You've got two good years left in you, Taylor," he said out of habit, the words mechanical. Then he paused, and something in his posture softened. "You really gonna quit now?"

Brett met his eyes. "It's not quitting," he said, steadier now. "I'm choosing my brain. I've done the research and I've listened to the players who came before me. I don't want to be another name on that list...I want to live a full life."

Coach Reynolds nodded slowly, the hard edge in his expression cracked just enough to show something deeper.

He stood up, stepped around the desk, and pulled Brett into a firm hug. His voice dropped to a whisper.

"Damn proud of you, boy...gonna miss you, Taylor."

After Brett left his office, Reynolds allowed himself to feel the relief. Brett had made it out. And this time, the ending wouldn't be a funeral.

Brett's Next Chapter

He didn't have a plan yet.

Walking away from football felt like stepping into a different kind of fog. The future was uncertain, and for the first time in years, Brett had no playbook to follow.

But he knew one thing...staying would have cost him everything.

That alone made the unknown worth facing.

He'd spent years being the player everyone expected him to be. Now, he had a chance to figure out who he really was beyond the helmet and beyond the game.

And even though he didn't know what would come next, he

finally had the space to find out.

And finally experienced something he'd been missing…hope.

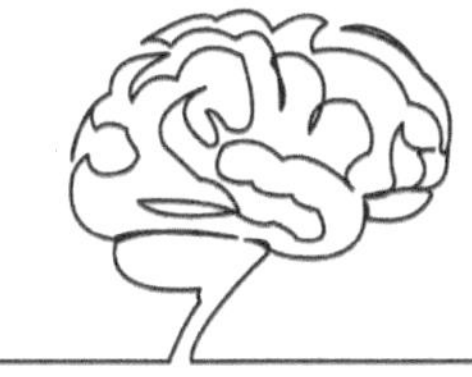

Walking Away Isn't Failure

Choosing to retire early is not weakness. It is one of the bravest acts an athlete can make.

> **Walking away means taking control.**
>
> **It means valuing your life beyond the scoreboard.**
>
> **It means protecting the only brain you get.**

'Walking away isn't quitting.
It's choosing yourself over a system that too often forgets the human cost.

Closing Reflection

Three perspectives marked Brett's turning point:

> **Brett:** Terrified of failure but resolute in choosing his brain over the game.

Angela: Relieved to see her son take control, ready to fight alongside him.

Marcus: Struggling to understand but facing the truth that toughness wasn't the only measure of manhood.

The crowd would never cheer for this moment. But it was the hardest choice, and the most important one, Brett Taylor would ever make.

Brett's Hidden Record

Total Hits (Games + Practices): 3,100

Unknown Concussions (Not Reported): 18 (Suspected)

Known / Reported Concussions: 2

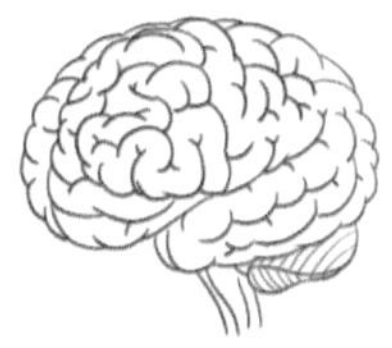

Fourth Quarter
Legacy & Reckoning

Kickoff

Football games are remembered for their fourth quarters. The last drive and final push. That moment where everything built across the game demands its price.

For Brett Taylor, the fourth quarter didn't happen under stadium lights, it began the day he walked away.

He had given seven years of his life to a sport that rewarded his toughness but punished his silence. He had collected thousands of hits, ignored countless symptoms, and carried expectations that were never truly his own. Now, the helmet was off and the field was behind him.

This quarter would be about what comes after, the life athletes are rarely taught to prepare for.

The whistle blew. The Fourth Quarter began and this time it was about Brett's future, his family, and the legacy of every hit that had brought him here.

What Remains

(Fourth Quarter Begins)

The helmet was gone, but Brett Taylor's fight was far from over.

Walking away from football had felt like losing everything: his identity, his scholarship and his future. The silence after the game was loud. For weeks, he sank under waves of guilt, shame, and depression. He felt like he'd let his teammates down, disappointed his coach, and failed his family. Without football, for the first time since he was twelve, Brett didn't know who he was.

But slowly, he began to rebuild.

Through his university's resources, Brett was referred to the on campus speech and language clinic. He worked with a speech-language pathologist (SLP) who specialized in cognitive rehabilitation.

Brett quickly realized that SLPs treat way more than just speech. They worked on improving his memory, attention, executive function, and so much more. They practiced strategies to manage the brain fog which helped alleviate his headaches. Honestly, it seemed like they were playing brain games more than anything else.

After a while, speech therapy stopped being hard and started being fun. Something he actually looked forward to.

One day in a session, she asked him a simple question: "*What do you want to do now?*"

Brett hesitated because he didn't know. For so long, football had been his only focus but her question stuck with him.

He also began seeing a neuro-optometrist, who retrained his vision, helping to reduce the stabbing glare of classroom lights and blurred text on the page.

A vestibular therapist drilled him through balance exercises that left him dizzy at first but gradually restored his physical stability.

Brett also began meeting with a mental health counselor, someone who helped him confront the depression that had been creeping in since high school. In those quiet sessions, he could be honest as he unpacked the weight of walking away. He was free to express the guilt and the fear of never being anything more than "the kid who quit."

And in doing that work, something unexpected began to surface: a new direction.

Brett started reading about cybersecurity. What started as curiosity, quickly turned to passion. It was a world of risk, protection and pattern recognition. The same discipline and focus he once poured into game film now fueled late-night study sessions and virtual labs. For the first time in a long time, Brett felt a new kind of purpose.

It took an extra year to graduate.
He didn't care. Every step forward was worth it.

The Fourth Quarter was about recovery, resilience, and reclaiming a future that football alone could never guarantee.

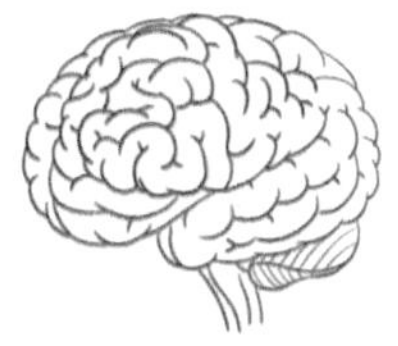

Chapter 10
New Dreams

Brett

The first time Brett walked into his cybersecurity class, he was nervous, reminiscent of the same adrenaline that once surged before kickoff. Only now, instead of turf and helmets, he faced screens filled with code.

No band. No scoreboard. No roar of the crowd.

But there was something else: possibility.

At first, he felt like a relic, older than most, carrying a redshirted year like a scar. The voice in his head hissed: *You failed. You quit. You're behind.*

But then he remembered the work he'd done in speech therapy. So another voice rose, steadier and clearer: *You chose your brain. You chose your life. And that's worth more than any trophy.*

Cybersecurity was really interesting to Brett. Every breach scenario, lit a familiar fire. It was strategy and defense. It was like a game but this time, the stakes were systems and not scoreboards.

Brett realized he made the right decision during a class hack-a-thon when he spotted a vulnerability no one else had noticed. His professor told him he had "the kind of thinking that stops real-world attacks," Brett smiled and exhaled with relief.

That was it. That was the moment.

He belonged.

When classmates asked about his past, Brett didn't hesitate to share, "Yeah, I played ball. But now I'm into cybersecurity." There was no shame, only truth.

He wasn't just the kid who walked away.

He was Brett Taylor, a student, a problem-solver and a survivor.

The Parentals

Brett stared at his phone before pressing the green video icon on his screen. He had spent the morning rehearsing what to say. *Would they care? Would they fake it? Would they still wish he was playing?*

He took a deep breath and tapped the video icon.

Angela beamed when he shared the news about being awarded an academic scholarship.

"You did this, Brett. Not football. You."

Marcus let the silence stretch before saying, "I never thought I'd see the day you'd get excited about a classroom. But… I'm proud of you, son."

Bridgette rolled her eyes, but the grin betrayed her pride. "See? Told you brains matter more than brawn."

Braxton, still inseparable from his football, listened wide-eyed as Brett explained hacking simulations and layered defenses.

"That's kinda like defense, huh? Just on computers instead of a field."

"Exactly," Brett said. "Still takes strategy and toughness, it's just a different kind."

The entire family was proud of him, they saw a young man rewriting his future and owning it.

Coach Reynolds

Coach Reynolds saw the email on a Friday afternoon.

He almost deleted it, assuming it was another GPA report or a last-minute schedule change.

But something made him open it.

Brett Taylor had officially withdrawn from football, declared a cybersecurity major,

and was on track to graduate.

Reynolds sat back.

He'd spent decades preaching toughness, teaching athletes to shake it off and push through. Brett changed the play when he decided to run a different route and choose something else.

And Reynolds couldn't help but wonder, was that the win he'd been missing all along?

He clicked out of the email, but didn't leave his desk.

Instead, he opened a browser and typed: "CTE symptoms in college athletes."

The screen filled with studies, interviews and warnings. He read stories that sounded all too familiar.

He scrolled for hours.

Then pulled out next week's practice schedule.

He stared at the drills he'd run for years: full contact days, no-pad Fridays and live scrimmage blocks.

And after 15 years of coaching, he questioned them.

He grabbed his playbook, picked up his pen and started crossing things out.

Reynold's swapped live hits for agility added time for film review and built in rest breaks he used to mock.

It wasn't much.

But it was something.

It was a start.

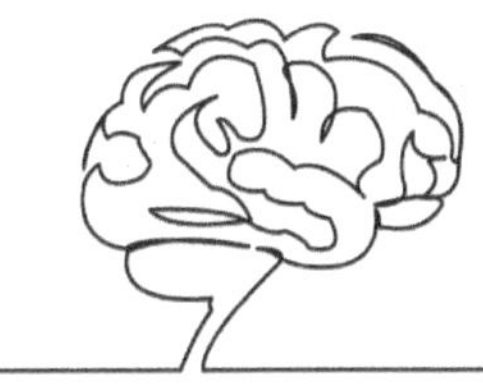

Reframing Identity Post-Sports

For many athletes, sports becomes the core of their identity. When the game ends, they feel lost and unsure of who they are without it.

Reframing identity means:

- Recognizing that skills like discipline, teamwork, and resilience transcend sport.
- Exploring new passions that align with those strengths.
- Understanding that walking away doesn't erase your legacy, it expands it.

Athletes are more than the sport they play.

Closing Reflection

Three perspectives witnessed Brett's transformation:

Brett: Igniting the same competitive fire in the cybersecurity arena.

His Family: Watching him stand taller but this time as a thinker and a builder.

Coach Reynolds: Redefining what it meant to be tough.

The stadium lights had faded.

But a new field had opened.

And Brett Taylor was already running full speed toward it.

Brett's Hidden Record

Total Hits (Games + Practices): 3,100

Unknown Concussions (Not Reported): 18 (Suspected)

Known / Reported Concussions: 2

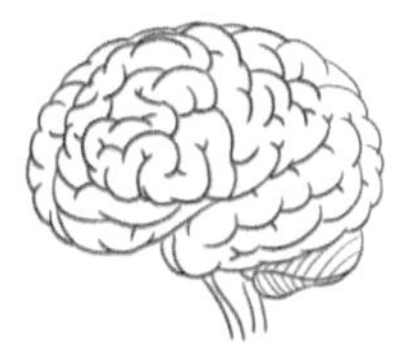

Chapter 11
The Assembly

Brett

The gymnasium of Brett's old high school smelled like sweat and floor polish, like familiar ghosts from another life. Brett stood just off the court, with notes in hand and his heart pounding louder than any drumline.

He used to come alive under lights like these. Now, they felt like interrogation lamps.

What if they don't listen? What if I choke? What if I'm still that kid who walked away?

He stepped to the podium anyway.

Rows of teenage athletes sat in folding chairs, with their jerseys on and awaiting the start of the assembly. Brett cleared his throat to speak.

"When I was your age, I thought things like headaches, dizziness, and mood swings were just part of the game," he began. "I thought if I said anything, I'd lose my spot and I thought toughness meant silence."

The students' heads tilted and their eyes locked in.

Brett told them about everything from the lights blurring into stars, to his collapse on the field. He also talked about the brain fog that turned classes into static, his denial and the cost.

Then, he told them the truth.

"Football taught me discipline and resilience," Brett said. "But the greatest lesson I ever learned was this…"

He paused for a moment before continuing. "You only get one brain. So, protect it. Don't be afraid to speak up. Take it from me, there's no trophy, scholarship or championship that is worth your future."

The gym was still. Everyone was focused on Brett.

He glanced up, quickly scanned the crowd to find his parents seated in the back and smiled.

It was in that moment, Brett saw it clearly.

His legacy wasn't on the field, it was here among the dozens of wide-eyed young athletes.

If Brett could teach one of those athletes to advocate for themselves, they may have the chance to walk away before it's too late.

Brett concluded the assembly with a quote from Dr. Kelli, "I'm not trying to stop you from playing, but I am here to raise your awareness and provide you with helpful information. Do with it what you will."

The Parentals

Angela sat near the back, tears pooling in her eyes with a pride that felt deeper than any victory dance. Every word her son spoke was healing, for him and for every parent listening.

Marcus sat beside her, arms folded but jaw clenched, his eyes were fixed on Brett. For years, he'd measured pride in grit and touchdowns. Tonight, he measured it in truth.

Bridgette nudged Braxton and whispered, "This is bigger than football."

Braxton, for once, didn't argue.

"Yeah," he whispered back. "This is so epic."

Coach Reynolds

Coach Reynolds had been digging.

It started when a former assistant sent him a video of Brett Taylor, standing at a high school podium, talking to young athletes about CTE.

The same kid Reynolds once told to "walk it off", was now warning others not to.

Something in his gut twisted.

He watched the movie *Concussion.*
Read about Mike Webster's descent.
Sat through the *Aaron Hernandez* documentaries, uneasy the whole time.

League of Denial left him staring at a blank screen long after the credits.

He pulled studies from the Center for Disease Control (CDC), National Collegiate Athletic Association (NCAA), and the National Institutes of Health (NIH).

Reynolds even signed up for a concussion certification course.

Maybe he couldn't fix the past, but he could open his eyes and prepare for a smarter future.

At practice, he stood on the sideline like always.

But now, he was watching differently.

A sophomore defensive back took a clean hit in a drill, shook his head, then slowly got up, off-balance and blinking too much.

Reynolds tracked him for a few steps. Recalling what he had learned about SHAAKE*.

He called him over.

"You didn't walk straight," he said.

"I tripped over a bag," the player lied, eyes darting toward the next rep.

"Don't lie to me," Reynolds said quietly. "I saw your eyes. Now, go see the trainer."

---

*Let's define SHAAKE: Spontaneous Headshake After a Kinematic Event A sudden, involuntary head shake that happens right after a hit or rapid head movement. Studies show this could be a potential sign of concussion.

The player hesitated.

"I said, now," he said low and deliberate through gritted teeth.

"Tell'em what happened and don't even think about watering it down."

The player finally nodded and jogged off, slower than before.

That night, Reynolds opened his laptop and created a new folder labeled "Smart Football".

Inside it, he dropped everything: articles, course links, quotes, stats and Brett's speech.

He didn't know exactly where this was going and that didn't matter.

Reynolds was determined to not only build a team but to protect it.

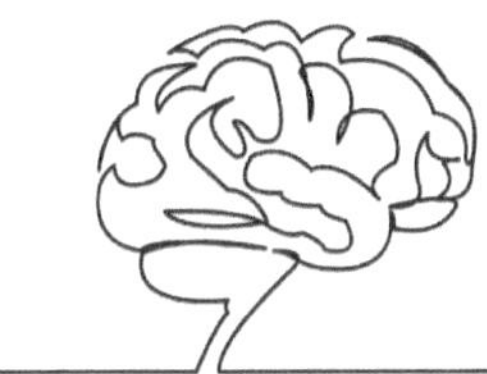

How Knowledge Spreads Impact

Awareness is contagious. When one athlete speaks the truth, it echoes beyond the gym.

Athletes listen to athletes.
Lived experience speaks louder than stats.

Stories shift culture.
They give others permission to speak.

Knowledge multiplies.
One honest voice can protect hundreds of futures.

The more truth we tell, the more lives we save.

Closing Reflection

Three perspectives revealed the new definition of success:

Brett: No longer chasing trophies but planting seeds of truth.

The Parentals: Watching their son rise.

Coach Reynolds: Learning that the best wins leave no one broken behind.

Brett's Hidden Record

Total Hits (Games + Practices): 3,100

Unknown Concussions (Not Reported): 18 (Suspected)

Known / Reported Concussions: 2

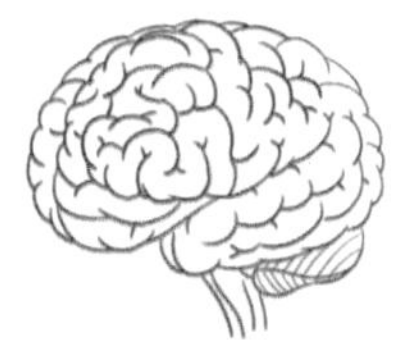

Chapter 12
The 25,000 Mark

Brett

The auditorium erupted in applause as Brett Taylor stepped across the stage.

"Brett Taylor, Bachelor of Science in Cybersecurity, cum laude."

For a flicker of a second, Brett imagined the glare of stadium lights, the deafening roar of a crowd, and his name booming across a football field.

But this? This was different.

This was earned. Brick by brick. This was a future he had built with resilience, grit, and a hundred hard choices no one had ever cheered for.

At 23, Brett finally understood the meaning of victory.

And it had nothing to do with scoreboards.

The Parentals

Angela clapped hard until her fingers were numb as tears streaming down her cheeks.

She remembered the nights she prayed he'd live to see this day.

Pride swelled in her chest so fiercely it hurt.

Marcus, stood beside Angela clapping, then leaned in and yelled over the cheers, "That's our son!"

His voice cracked on the last word.

For the first time, he understood that Brett's toughness hadn't ended with football, it had just changed form.

Bridgette and Braxton leapt to their feet, cheering louder than anyone.

For Bridgette, this degree represented a moment…years ago… when a little sister stood up and said, *"This matters."*

A Brother and Sister

That evening, after the photos and toasts and hugs, Brett stepped onto the balcony of the family's rented house near campus.

Bridgette was already there, standing poised with her hands placed on the balcony railing looking up at the stars. Now she was taller and older but still had the same no-nonsense stare that had once cracked open everything.

"Hey, Bridge," he said softly.
She turned, her grin already forming. "Hey, college graduate."

Brett rubbed the back of his neck. The words caught in his throat before they even formed. But he pushed them out, because they mattered.

"In a way… you saved my life."

He swallowed hard. "If I hadn't come home that day and if you hadn't made me listen, I don't know where I'd be. Honestly, I don't think I'd even be here. I don't think I'd be… at all."

Tears welled in his eyes. He blinked them back. They fell anyway.

Bridgette stepped forward, stood on her tippy toes, and wrapped her arms around him. His shoulders shook as he buried his face in her hair.

She whispered, "Thanks for listening." Then, quieter,

"I love you, big brother."

"I love you too," Brett whispered back, voice breaking.

And there, beneath the quiet sky, they stood, as survivors of a moment that changed everything.

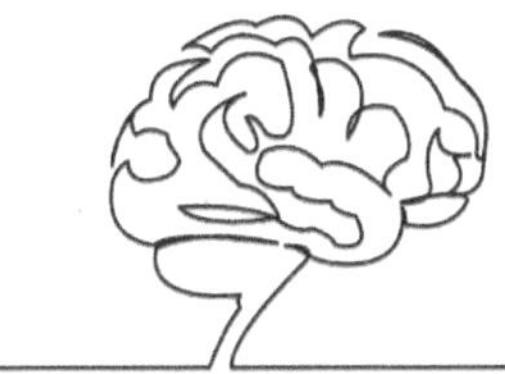

Every Hit Matters, Every Choice Matters More

To Athletes: Your body and brain are your future. Protect them. No game, scholarship, or trophy are worth your life.

To Parents: Trust your instincts. Push for answers. Don't minimize the signs, act on them.

To Coaches: Your words and your actions shape the culture. Encourage honesty. Build trust. Winning isn't everything.

Closing Reflection

The final whistle had blown on Brett Taylor's football career. But his life was just beginning.
He wasn't defined by tackles, or hits, or broken helmets.

He was defined by the moment he chose his brain.
By the sister who spoke up.
By the legacy he dared to build from scratch.

The 25,000 Mark wasn't just a number.
It was a truth. A warning. A reckoning.
And ultimately, a beginning.

Brett Taylor had learned the hardest lesson:
You only get one brain.

And with his, he would build a future worth protecting.

Brett's Hidden Record

Total Hits (Games + Practices): 3,100

Unknown Concussions (Not Reported): 18 (Suspected)

Known / Reported Concussions: 2

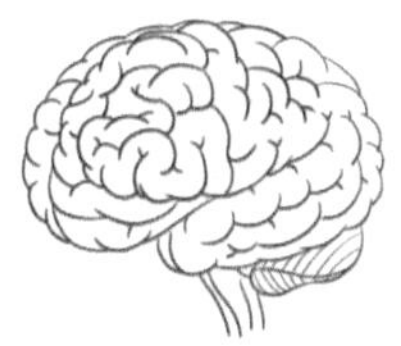

Conclusion
The 25,000 Mark

Brett Taylor was one of the fortunate ones. He had awareness, access to care, and most of all, a mom and baby sister who refused to give up on him. Bridgette's spark of truth lit the path that changed everything. Thanks to her, Brett never reached the 25,000 mark. He stopped short, walked away, and reclaimed his life.

After graduation, Brett accepted a position in cybersecurity with a starting salary in the six figures. The paycheck was proof of his hard work, but the real reward was deeper. Brett felt like Brett again. He was able to laugh more, his mood swings faded and he became fun again. Brett was back to being the brother Bridgette and Braxton remembered from before the fog.

Brett's story didn't end on the field. It continued in classrooms, auditoriums, and communities. Through his advocacy and determination to give back, he partnered with the Brain Talk Foundation to continue raising awareness. He stood on stages, spoke at schools, and shared his journey at Brain Talk Day. The same event where Bridgette first learned about the egg-and-yolk analogy that opened his eyes years before.

But Brett knew not every athlete was so fortunate. Too many never hear the truth in time. Too many keep playing, keep hitting, and keep ignoring the signs until it's too late. Some face dementia in their twenties, thirties and beyond. Others lose their lives to CTE before they ever get the chance to heal. Brett Taylor lived because knowledge reached him. His life became proof that awareness, love, and courage can change the story.

The 25,000 Mark is much more than a number. it's a warning and a wake-up call. Every hit matters. But so do the choices made after the hits. Brett's choice was to stop, to heal, and to live. And because of that, his story continues.

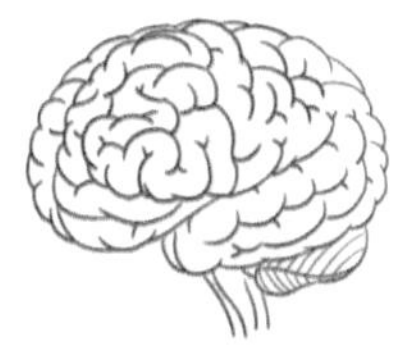

Epilogue
Beyond the 25,000 Mark

Brett's story is a story of hope. But it is not the story for everyone.

Too many athletes never hear the truth in time. Too many parents don't know the signs and too many coaches reinforce silence instead of safety.

The cost is devastating:

> Athletes showing signs of dementia as early as their twenties.
>
> Families grieving sons and daughters lost to suicide.
>
> Generations of athletes carrying invisible injuries no trophy can outweigh.

That is why education matters. That is why advocacy matters. That is why you matter.

> **To Athletes:** You are more than your sport. Protect your brain. Speak up.
>
> **To Parents:** Never ignore the warning signs. Trust your instincts. Push for answers. One conversation could save your child's future.

To Coaches: Redefine toughness. Create a culture where honesty is honored, not punished. You have the power to protect your players beyond the game.

Brett's partnership with the **Brain Talk Foundation** became his way of giving back. Through school visits, Brain Talk Day events, and public advocacy, he used his second chance to ignite awareness in others.

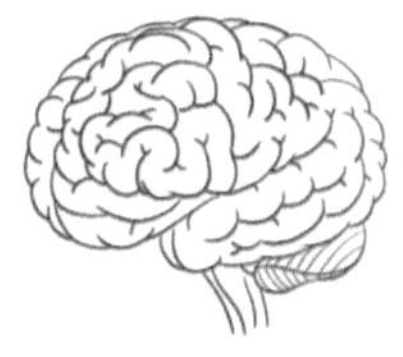

Reader's Reflection
Your 25,000 Mark

Brett Taylor's story is fictional, but the risks of concussion, TBI, and CTE are very real. His journey shows that every hit matters, every symptom matters, and every choice matters. Now it's your turn to reflect.

For Athletes

Have you ever "shaken off" a hit instead of reporting it?

What fears keep you from speaking up about your symptoms?

How can you redefine toughness to include protecting your brain?

For Parents

What warning signs would you look for if your child played sports?

How would you respond if your child told you they were struggling with headaches, memory, or mood?

What conversations can you start now to ensure your child feels safe speaking up?

For Coaches & Educators

How do you define toughness for your players or students?

What messages do you send, directly or indirectly, about reporting injuries?

What steps can you take to create a safer culture on your team or in your school?

Takeaway: Everyone has a role in preventing brain injury and protecting futures. The question is, what will your role be?

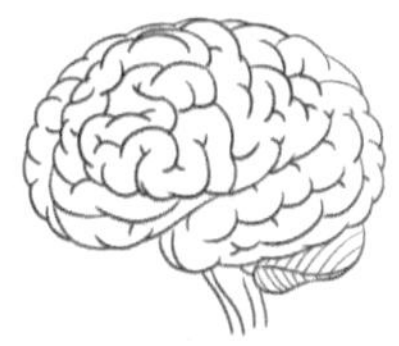

Glossary of Terms

The 25,000 Mark

This symbolic threshold is inspired by a statement from Dr. Bennet Omalu, the forensic pathologist who first identified CTE in the brain of former NFL player Mike Webster. In describing the extent of Webster's brain trauma, Dr. Omalu equated it to surviving **25,000 car crashes**. While there is no definitive number of head impacts that causes CTE, the 25,000 mark represents an urgent warning—a wake-up call to the cumulative danger of repeated hits, especially in youth athletes. In this story, the 25,000 mark serves as a metaphor for the invisible line that, once crossed, may change everything.

Brain Talk Day

A real, annual event hosted by the Brain Talk Foundation, a nonprofit organization committed to educating communities, schools, and families about brain health, concussion awareness, and CTE prevention. Brain Talk Day features speakers, workshops, and storytelling designed to spark critical conversations around youth sports and brain safety.

CTE (Chronic Traumatic Encephalopathy)

A progressive and often fatal brain disease caused by repeated head impacts. CTE can lead to symptoms such as memory loss, emotional instability, depression, aggression, and dementia. It can only be definitively diagnosed after death.

Concussion

A mild form of traumatic brain injury that results from a bump, blow, or jolt to the head or body, causing the brain to move rapidly inside the skull. Symptoms may include headaches, dizziness, confusion, nausea, fatigue, and sensitivity to light or sound.

Concussion Protocol

A set of procedures followed when an athlete is suspected of having a concussion. It typically includes immediate removal from play, medical evaluation, and a gradual return-to-play timeline.

"The Fog"

A non-medical phrase used by individuals recovering from brain injuries to describe mental confusion, difficulty concentrating, memory lapses, emotional swings, or a sense of detachment.

Kandid Konversations with Dr. Kelli

A podcast hosted by Dr. Kelli Dunham, founder of the Brain Talk Foundation. The show features open, honest dialogue with athletes, parents, medical professionals, and advocates about brain health, sports culture, and the real-life impact of TBIs.

Through storytelling and candid insight, the podcast expands on the themes explored in this book.

PCS (Post-Concussion Syndrome)
An older term used to describe when symptoms from a concussion last longer than expected. These symptoms may include headaches, trouble focusing, memory problems, mood changes, and sleep issues. PCS is often used when symptoms continue for about three months or longer in adults.

PPCS (Persistent Post-Concussive Symptoms)

A more current term used to describe ongoing symptoms after a concussion. Most people recover within a few weeks. When symptoms last longer than four weeks in youth or longer than three months in adults, they are called persistent post-concussive symptoms (PPCS).

This term is preferred because it focuses on symptoms that can improve over time, rather than suggesting a permanent condition. PPCS can affect daily life, including school, work, and relationships.

Return-to-Play Protocol
A medically supervised step-by-step process that determines when an athlete can safely return to practice or competition following a concussion. Skipping steps increases the risk of serious injury.

Second Impact Syndrome

A rare but dangerous condition that occurs when a second concussion is sustained before the first one has fully healed. It can lead to rapid brain swelling and, in many cases, death.

SHAAKE

An acronym for "Spontaneous Headshake After a Kinematic Event," a sudden, involuntary head shake that occurs right after a hit or rapid head movement.

Subconcussive Hits

Repeated impacts to the head that do not cause noticeable symptoms at the time but may still cause cumulative brain damage over time. These are common in contact sports and often go unreported.

TBI (Traumatic Brain Injury)

A disruption in normal brain function caused by a blow or jolt to the head. TBIs can range from mild (like concussions) to severe and can affect thinking, memory, mood, and behavior long-term.

Acknowledgements

First and foremost, I thank God for the vision, the strength, and the purpose to do this work.

To my parents, thank you for your unwavering love, support, and belief in the prototype.

To my family, Sorors, and friends, thank you for loving me through the process and for encouraging me when it was heavy.

To my phenomenal Brain Talk team, thank you for walking beside me in this mission. Your dedication, passion, and commitment to changing lives do not go unnoticed.

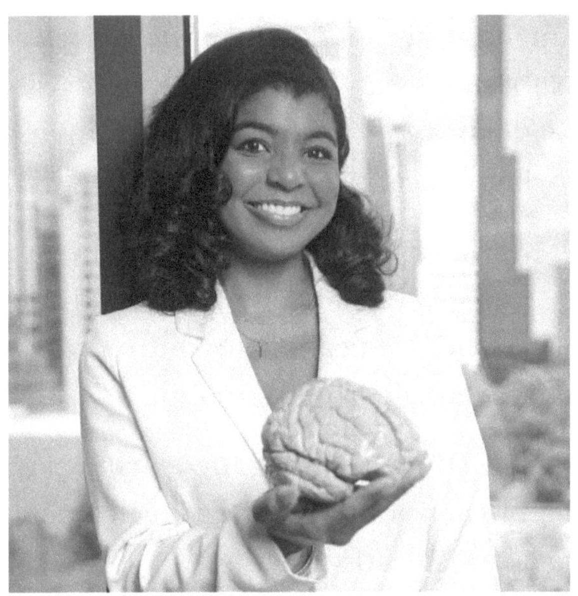

About The Author

Dr. Kelli A. Uitenham is an assistant clinical professor at Northeastern University's Charlotte campus, a TEDxCharlotte speaker, keynote presenter, and founder of the Brain Talk Foundation, a nonprofit organization committed to raising awareness around concussion, traumatic brain injury (TBI), and chronic traumatic encephalopathy (CTE) through education, outreach, and storytelling.

She is also the owner of a private telepractice focused on providing accessible, evidence-based care and consultation in brain health and communication disorders. Through her clinical work, academic leadership, and nonprofit advocacy, Dr. Uitenham empowers individuals, families, and communities to protect their futures, one informed decision at a time.

Dr. Uitenham hosts the podcast *Kandid Konversations with Dr. Kelli*, where she leads bold, honest conversations with athletes, parents, educators, and experts about brain injuries, sports culture, and what it means to truly put health first.

The 25,000 Mark is her debut novel, a fictional narrative grounded in truth. Inspired by real lives and urgent realities, the book reflects her dedication to shifting the conversation around youth sports, safety, and strength.

When she's not writing, speaking, or teaching, Dr. Uitenham continues her mission to make brain health personal, and to ensure that awareness leads to action.

Learn more at www.braintalkfoundation.org

Listen to the podcast by search *Kandid Konversations with Dr. Kelli* on your favorite streaming platforms.

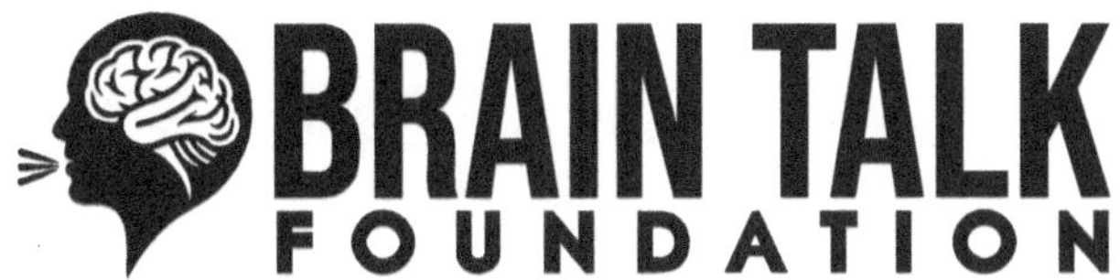

Visit us @ BrainTalkFoundation.org

Brain Talk Foundation is dedicated to raising awareness and educating communities about concussions, traumatic brain injuries (TBI), and chronic traumatic encephalopathy (CTE).

Support the Mission

Your donation helps us continue
raising awareness and serving communities:
www.braintalkfoundation.org

Bring Brain Talk to You

Interested in booking Dr. Kelli for a speaking engagement?
Visit our website to learn more and submit an inquiry.

Listen & Learn

Kandid Konversations with Dr. Kelli
Real conversations, expert insight, and stories that matter.
Available on all major streaming platforms.

Stay Connected

@braintalkfoundation | @drkellibraintalkslp

www.ingramcontent.com/pod-product-compliance
Lightning Source LLC
LaVergne TN
LVHW051011080826
845145LV00009B/2565